When health is absent, wisdom cannot reveal itself, art cannot become manifest, strength cannot be exerted, wealth is useless and reason is powerless.

Hemophilis, 300BC

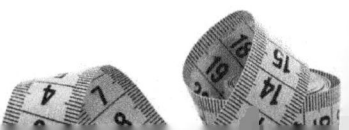

INTRODUCTION

The purpose of this book is to give you information about weight management and to answer the questions that people most frequently ask when they try to lose weight. This is an unbiased guide, not for the benefit of any company or industry. It is information for you to use when you are interested in losing weight.

In order for us to understand obesity and being overweight, we need to know the definition according to World Health Organization (WHO). They say it is an extra accumulation of fat in our body that causes health problems. Basically this means you have excess fat in your body, additional fat tissue which eventually will make you sick.

Being overweight accounts for about 60% of the health care costs in the United States, Mexico, and all other countries. Diabetes is on the rise, as is cardiovascular disease and cancer. A very good chunk of all healthcare costs are put into these three.

In the United States, one in three men are on some type of diet trying to lose weight.

Two in three females are on some type of diet to lose weight.

It seems like everybody knows what to do, but nobody is getting the long-term results.

For the past 20 years, cases of being overweight or obese have at least doubled, or even tripled.

Obesity in the United States is considered an illness; it officially has an ICD-9 code.

The number one cause of death in Mexico and the United

States is cardiovascular disease. Without doubt, Mexico and the United States have the highest incidence of diabetes, and in Mexico 37.5% of the total population is obese. In the United States, 35.7% of the total population is obese. This is not counting people that are overweight.

According to the CDC in the United States, 17% of the kids 2 to 18 are obese. This is a serious concern because for a lot of these kids the future is uncertain because of their health. I have personally seen kids as young as 12 years old with high pressure. Another common serious issue is hypoglycemia in teenagers. This is no longer a cosmetic issue; it is a major crisis in healthcare.

Between the ages 2 and 5, the amount of over weight kids has been decreasing. The total is 13.5% in the United States, which is still very high. Unfortunately, the statistics for Hispanics and African American young men are higher.

The facts are presented not to scare you, but for you to act on. This issue is cutting your life in half and you are not enjoying your life to its fullness. When you are not one hundred percent, you cannot act 100%. In fact, losing weight is simple, easy and painless if you get the right information from the right source. The problem here is that so many people are benefiting from your pain; it's time for you to act smart, get the right information, get the right tools and fight back with knowledge.

For most of the people that have extra weight, it translates into becoming diabetic. Diabetes type II is on the rise as well, and only 12% of the diabetic population have the illness under control. In the United States alone, it is believed that 60% of the population is diabetic, pre-diabetic, or already has hypoglycemia. This disease alone can literally destroy your body over time. Most of the patients I have seen have issues with their hair, their teeth, their skin, their main organs such as kidneys, liver, heart, eyes, and lower extremities--it's called neuropathies.

The obesity problem is very lucrative for some industries. For example, two billion dollars goes to the fitness industry, and we don't even talk about healthcare system being a $1 trillion industry. And   remember what I said before, that 60% of the cost is caused by being overweight or obese. My approach to this problem is to start taking control of your own health and your body, because at the end of the day you are the one paying extra money, and also you are the one suffering.

This guide will show you the most frequent questions from my patients and clients. The answers will be in simple every-day, common language, and sometimes we will refer to a client patient and tell you their story to make an explanation easy.

So let's get ready.

Get Free Guides:
1.-Are you craving movement
2.- 10 Tips To Lose Weight
3.-Coffee 10 quick Perks

www.healthyhappythinanddietfree.com
Text the word dietfree to 58885

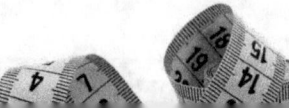

The Doctor of The Future will give no medicine but will interest his patients in the care of the human frame, in diet and in cause and prevention of disease.

Thomas Edison.

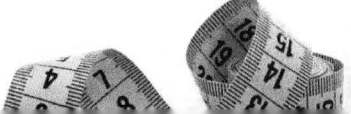

CHAPTER 1

Why am I doing this?

Ever since I was a little girl, my passion was medicine. As far back as I can remember, I used to play with my dad. I was the doctor and he was my patient My dad played that game with me until I was 13 or 14 years old. Maybe my passion came from the struggle with my own health. I was always sick when I was kid. Twice I almost didn't make it-- you know what I mean. At one point the doctors informed my parents that I only had a few hours to live. I know what being sick is, and I know how important it is to be healthy.

When I first went to college, I studied agricultural engineering. I don't know if my passion had died around that time or if I just did not want to follow it.

But when you have a purpose in life, things are always going to fall in place no matter what you do, in order for you to fulfill your destiny. It's not magic, you have to follow a path. I learned this the hard way when my younger kid got sick.

My child was only one year old. It was three days   after his birthday. I remember clearly that they took him for his first year's checkup and his shots one day before his birthday. Three days later, his lymph nodes swelled to the point that it was noticeable from afar.
I took him to the pediatrician right away. The first thing that she told me was, "I don't know what this child has, but it is something really serious, so you had better admit him into the hospital."

Right away my reaction was denial. I didn't want to hear that. I immediately took him to another doctor who told me the same thing. I took him to five pediatricians in total before he was admitted into the hospital.

In the hospital, for the first month it was a roller coaster. One day they said he had cancer, another day they said tuber ulosis, then leukemia--all the awful diseases they suspected he had.

After a month, doctors came to talk to me and said that they knew what he had. Its name is Hystiocitosis. After they left I felt a kind of relief because I didn't know what it was. I thought it was only for a day, like a cold. Then the next day the doctors brought me a lot of literature to read about the illness. Well it turned out to be something really serious, an autoimmune disorder.

Hystiocytosis is rare condition. It happens to one in 1 million. I was so mad, because I felt like God was counting and pointed at my kid and he said, "You're one million. Here, I give you this illness." I was mad because my child isn't supposed to be sick, my kid was wanted, always well taken care of. I don't drink, I don't smoke, I never use drugs. He was breast fed and always ate very healthy. There was no reason for my kid to get sick. It is awful to see your kid going to chemotherapy, to see all the procedures that they do to him, to see that your kid is looking into your eyes, begging you for help.

My kid was in the hospital almost as an impatient for around one year after that. It was hard to do anything besides be by his side in the hospital. At one point I got so mad that I decided never to pray again.

Since conventional doctors didn't have an answer, I decided to take matters into my own hands. I went back to school to study Naturopathic medicine, Oriental medicine, hypnosis and nutrition, trying to find something to help my child. Believe me, it wasn't easy because I already had my three kids and husband and had to work. My kids were little and the main stream of income was mine. But I needed to help my child. That was my main concern back then. I tried everything with him: Oriental medicine herbs, homeopathic medicine, acupuncture, flower essence, nutrition and even implemented some lifestyle changes.

For me, ever since the beginning of my journey of seeing Patients, my goal was finding an answer for my own child, learning as much as I can. I always gave a hundred percent when I was treating each patient. In school they said that some patients followed you more than others. The patient following ever since my internship had diabetes, pain, and weight management problems. At the beginning it was hard for me because I didn't understand the problem. It seemed so easy when they explained it to me in school: it's all about calories.

I have to admit that I never had any problem with weight, so because I didn't experience the problem I thought it was very easy to solve--not at all! My typical recommendation was eat fewer calories and increase exercise. Some people get results at the beginning, and then a month later or two months later they're back at square one, frustrated. In some cases, when I went to the front desk to check some paperwork, when my patients were there for weight management, I found them hiding what they were eating, things such as candy, soda, or bakery. Also I found that people were lying to me when it was time for intake. So I didn't understand what was going on. To me it was like if you want to lose weight, you're going to do everything you need to do in order for you to lose weight. But in reality this is not true. I became for them the food Police Department.

If you know me by now, you know that have to come back with something. My approach was to take more classes such as hypnotherapy, nutrition, courses related to weight management, books, enroll in tons of e-courses. I studied over 100 diets to make sense out of it. After all this nonsense, it clicked. I had the answer all along: it was doing the same thing that I was doing all my life. It works; I was proof of it.

This is what I found out: Diets don't work. You need less exercise than everybody's saying you do. There are five different causes for gaining weight; food and exercise is not the only answer. For this reason I want to make sure that you understand these causes. I'm going to address a lot of questions that you have in the back of your mind. Many of these concepts you will not find anywhere else.

Most of my clients and patients need a complete program, not just parts and pieces or make-believe. I also found out that a lot of people were doing some dangerous procedures that can have serious negative side effects. This is the main thing which is important for you to know, how you can do it safely, improve your health, improve your appearance and feel excellent.

My ideal results would be that everyone who gets into my programs becomes healthy, happy, thin without diets, and to get these results permanently. Losing weight is easy if you have the right concepts and if you have the right teacher.

Get Free Guides:
1.-Are you craving movement
2.- 10 Tips To Lose Weight
3.-Coffee 10 quick Perks

www.healthyhappythinanddietfree.com
Text the word dietfree to 58885

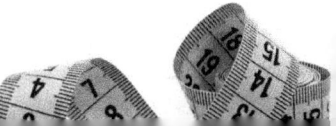

CHAPTER 2

One of the most frequent questions that people ask me is what is the best diet. My answer will be that no one else's diet works; the ideal diet is what you customize for yourself, using food and flavors that you like, making simple and easy changes.

Let me tell you a story of one of my clients. She came to me wanting to lose only 15 pounds. She told me it was literally impossible to do that because she already tried so many diets, she exercised, but she could not lose the extra weight. She even asked me if I like challenges, because she was herself a challenge. I told her that we can always try. Give me three months and we will see the results.

My approach to get fast and easy results was through food, but I knew that it was not a permanent solution; it was a bandit. In the second month I got into the emotional aspect of the problem and the stress management portion of it. She loves how my way works permanently, because after one and a half years she is keeping it up, she looks fantastic and she feels awesome.

At the beginning of all my programs, I do an intake to get a ballpark view on how to accommodate my clients. So many people never open up to you at the beginning, but asking them questions gets you a sense of where there are. That is where the beauty happens. Considering the complex nature of the human mind and body, we have to take an approach where we complement each other. You are not whole, but the approach for the solution has to be whole.

My client is a typical example of people focusing only on food, or bowing to a diet. She was making tons of mistakes about the food she was choosing. I even went the extra step--checking her pantry, explaining why each item should or shouldn't be there. She learned how to read labels and became aware of the terms that companies use to confuse you, the types of ingredients and the tricks. I can tell you for a fact that she's a success because she looks happier. She did not just lose that weight, she got her life back on her own terms. Now she has a better relationship with food, and she can enjoy food again.

This is one of the main reasons why I tell people that diets don't work, because you ruin the relationship between you and food. And this one is sacred, because we have to eat the rest of our lives.

Why do we need to eat food that we don't like, or a certain amount of food that makes us hungry all the time? These are two things that can hurt us in the long run.

If someone asks you what type of diet you are on, answer "(your name) diet", for example "Georgina's diet" for me. So go ahead, put your name on your diet and customize it for yourself.

One more question people often ask me is how many hours should I exercise each day. I'm going to disappoint you with this. According to sports medicine, it is recommended that you do two and a half hours of mild exercise a week, and one and a half hours of more intense exercise a week.

It is true the exercise has a lots of benefits. It can help you to reduce stress, to increase serotonin (which makes you feel happy), give you energy, reduce stiffness, improve cardiovascular disease, give you more flexibility, and also increase the amount of oxygen in your body.

The benefits are endless, but nobody's talking about the negative side effects of exercise. Also nobody talks about how you can transform exercise into something fun and productive.

I have noticed that people who do so much exercise have problems with their joints, pains, brain damage, and some deformities in certain places due to the excessive exercise that they perform. Incorporating exercise into your life can be fun as well; dancing can be fun, walking your dog, gardening, and also doing chores in your house. One of my major exercises is to spend time with my family by walking our dogs. It's a good time to talk, to enjoy nature, to relax and have some sanity in my home (dogs are very active). After we walk my dogs, my house is quiet, I can concentrate on work, I can be more productive and also feel good about it. This is one of the examples that you can take, for you to do some activities that you enjoy. According to Harvard University, 15 minutes of activity that you like will increase your happiness (meaning increase the production of serotonin in your brain).

Think of all the possibilities. What do you like? What extra activities can become a bigger part of your life? What fun things do you want to do and how can you incorporate them? Be creative-- the possibilities are endless.

Let me tell you story about one of my clients. He was a former professional hockey player, and he came to me for pain management. It was to the point that he was having trouble sleeping due to the pain. All of his injuries happened while he was playing hockey or training.

The treatment was for him use acupuncture. I also incorporated certain foods to reduce inflammation, which aids in alleviating pain. He got to the point that he could manage his pain and reduce the amount of medication that he was taking; he even sometimes managed without it.

How I can get rid of my belly fat?

Belly fat is one of the hardest things to get rid of. So many people lose muscle mass first, and even then sometimes never lose the belly fat.

Based on my experience, a lot of people have constipation. It's a frequent problem for so many of my patients that really have belly fat. For them it is normal to have a bowel movement every two or three days. I have to explain that if you eat three times, then they have to have three bowel move ments a day, not one every two or three days.

Some of my clients even mention that are interested in losing belly fat only, not from their breasts or booty. The last two are the most common areas to accumulate fat. But some programs that they do make them lose muscle mass, because they're doing it incorrectly.

So going back to how you can get rid of belly fat, here are some tips: balance insulin (one of the first symptoms of pre-diabetes is the big belly), increase the amount of live bacteria, get the proper amount of water, increase fiber intake, add some good fats into your diet, and reduce foods that can cause your constipation.

Recently I had a client who had hypoglycemia. She was overweight and had panic attacks. Because her condition was a little delicate, I helped her to balance insulin. She lost the belly fat, she lost weight, and she got rid of the panic attacks. This is only one technique that you can use to reduce belly fat. Another technique that you can use to reduce belly fat is to get into detox; most of my clients that go into detox lose belly fat automatically.

What food I can eat?

People want the magic behind everything, but there is no one food, no one pill, not one thing only, but a combination of foods that you need in order for you to keep that weight off. You have to remember that you need variety, flavors that you enjoy, the whole color spectrum. And yes, sometimes eat something that you're not supposed to in order to keep sanity into your life.

There is no such a thing as a magic food. It seems like that's what everybody's looking for; you have to be a smarter than that. If it is too good to be true, don't buy it. Remember the problem of obesity has been increasing in the last 50 years; you have to ask yourself what is the difference between how we live in today and how they lived 100 years ago? How was the food back then? How was the lifestyle back then? What were the types of ativity back then? What type of food they were eating?

How is this different from today? How you can improve your food base of knowledge?

You can be more creative about this topic, but remember you body is very complex and needs all sorts of nutrients.

I have some clients that are taking some herbs that contain caffeine. I will not recommend this because it can damage the adrenal glands and all of your endocrine system (hormones). As you know, the hormones in your body control the delivery of messages from brain to body. If you translate it, hormones mean messenger. In order for you to do any activity in with your body, your brain has to initiate it and send the info to the glands. These give the info to hormones. They deliver the message and then things happen in your body.

Another very common mistake is that people focus on one single thing to lose weight such as zero calorie foods like diet pop. Most of these products do not make you lose weight--to the contrary, they make you gain more weight over time because they make you eat more. You have to understand that your brain is very smart, so many of these products are all empty calories with no nutrients, so your brain is looking for the nutrients such as vitamins, minerals, fats, good carbohydrates and protein to function properly. And this is the reason why it makes you eat more, because you need certain things that you don't have in your body to function.

This is one of the main ways that people destroy their good

relationship with food, by eating one particular food only, and is also one of the main reasons why people never lose weight, and cheat all the time trying to lose weight.

Years ago my neighbor used to babysit kids, and my kids that were little would sometimes play with the kids that my neighbor babysat. One girl that used to play with my daughter also attended the same school as my kids. For Mexican people, the 15-year-old party is a big deal, and moms would always recommend that the girls lose weight to look their very best for their party. The girl took food supplements and was losing the weight extremely fast. She developed chronic anemia, and instead of having a birthday party they had a funeral. She did wear the dress that she was looking forward to wearing in the birthday party; she took it to her grave.

Like I said before, you need variety, different colors and good tasting foods for your taste buds.

Food is good for you, so keep a good relationship with food, and if it is too good to be true, doubt it.

How long is the diet for?

I don't know!
You have to understand that each case is different. Everybody's special and complex. It depends on how many pounds you need to lose, if you have any health problems that concern you, and also if you're willing to do the task.

I had a client that in six months lost 53 pounds. At the same time, another client lost 40 pounds in six months. The difference was the lifestyle and willingness. The one who lost 53 pounds had a purpose, and the other one was doing it just because. But I think the two of them were doing the right thing. Most of my clients lose at average about 1 to 2 pounds a week, and some weeks they lose nothing at all. My theory behind this is it's not how fast you get there, it's is staying there longer or even permanently. I do not promote programs that make you lose weight fast because that can damage your organs and have so many negative side effects. I had one of my clients lose weight with the Atkins diet. He overdid it; he lost in one month about 45 pounds. About a year later he ended up on dialysis. This is the main reason why I am careful what to promote.

Can I eat meat?

Yes, without doubt. This is a topic is very controversial for so many professional people in the field of nutrition and even some gurus.

If we use common sense, our body is equipped to eat meat. We have choleric acid in our digestive system and we have our back teeth to chew.

As far as the nutrients, remember no plants have vitamin B12, only blue-green algae and meat. The iron in plants is not good quality for your body to absorb, while meat on the other hand has very good quality iron.

This is one of the main reasons why so many vegetarians have anemia, because the supply of iron and B12 is not good quality. Another common missing nutrient is zinc.

I think the controversy started in how the animals are raised for slaughter. In the agriculture field you have to be productive in order for you to keep a business. You have a limited time to raise X animals; for example, pigs, six months; chickens, six weeks; cows, 12 months. If you leave the animals alive longer your profit is gone, and this is the main reason why people don't raise animals the oldfashioned way, because is not cost- effective.

Animals are forced to live in such a bad conditions, such as small dirty confined places. They have to use drugs such as vaccines and antibiotics for the farmer to be profitable, and also to have affordable food in our groceries. Remember grocery stores are another factor. The time there should be limited on the shelves, so they have to use chemicals (gases), or freeze their meat for years.

I will not recommend eating meat only. You will lose weight but you will get a lot of negative side effects as a consequence. My suggestion is at least keep 20 to 40% animal-based foods in your diet, and for the rest use plant-based foods.

If you can afford it, buy organic meat and keep the ratio 20-40 %. If you like meat enjoy it and be conscious of what type of farmers you support. If we make it a ritual eventually all of them will have to do the right thing for us, our health, and for the animals.

For some of my clients, the simple fact of being without meat is not doable, and we have to use a balanced approach to everything that we do and everything we eat.

Are fats so bad?

Most of my clients/patients are confused about fats. For centuries mankind has use fats for cooking. Even our brain is made of fat.

Here is the list of some good fats that we have been using for centuries; some of these aren't used in modern cooking because they are claimed to be bad: butter, tallow and suet from beef and lamb, lard from pigs, poultry fat, coconut, palm and palm kernel oils. For salads, use extra virgin olive oil (also OK for cooking), expeller-expressed sesame and peanut oils, expeller-expressed flax oil (in small amounts). For fat-soluble vitamins, use cod liver oil (preferable to fish oils, which do not provide fat-soluble vitamins, and can cause an overdose of unsaturated fatty acids and usually come from farmed fish.) You have to also remember about the good practices in the farms which make a huge difference in the quality of the fats. Not all of the newfangled fats (manmade) are good. Some are bad and can cause cancer, heart disease, immune system dysfunction, sterility, learning disabilities, growth problems and osteoporosis. Hydrogenated and partially hydrogenated oils, industrially processed liquid oils such as soy, corn, safflower, cottonseed and canola, fats and oils (especially vegetable oils) heated to very high temperatures in processing and frying can all be harmful.

It is recommended to eat fats as a form of producing energy, as a fuel generator, rather than to use grains for that purpose. Some fats are recommended to lose weight, such as the fat in avocados, fish oil, nuts and seeds to mention few. The idea of gaining weight when you eat fat is all schooling and it has been proved that it is wrong.

So my recommendation is add more fats into your daily diet, and reduce the intake of grains.

One fact: we are bombarded with radiation from electronics; butter has a component that can help you to protect your brain from radiation (real butter, good farm-raised chemical-free butter).

Fish oil can help you to unclog the arteries, and one of the side effects it has is making you smarter.

Coconut oil has been used for centuries as a skincare and for cooking. It is believed to have so many health benefits. Some experts claim that is good for cancer treatment.

Add more fats, increase the flavoring, move yourself forward and become smarter.

Recently, an editorial by Harvard's Walter Willett, M.D., in the American Journal of Public Health (1990) acknowledged that even though "the focus of dietary recommendations is usually a reduction of saturated fat intake, no relation between saturated fat intake and risk of CHD was observed in the most informative prospective study to date."

He further admitted that "...In Framingham, for example, we found that the people who ate the most cholesterol, ate the most saturated fat, ate the most calories, weighed the least, and were the most physically active."

It is not known exactly how much food made with lauric oils is needed in order to have a protective level of lauric acid in the diet. Infants probably consume between 0.3 and 1 gram per kilogram of body weight if they are fed human milk or an enriched infant formula that contains coconut oil. This amount appears to have always been protective. Adults could probably benefit from the consumption of 10 to 20 grams of lauric acid per day. Growing children probably need about the same amounts as adults.

Source: http://www.westonaprice.org

Types of exercises designed for weight loss

Any movement is better than no movement at all. The recommendation is for 2 1/2 hours of mild exercise and one and a half hours of intense exercise per week.

I just want to remind you of something. If you don't exercise for one year, what would happen? Maybe you will lose same muscle mass, and your muscle will become more jiggly, that's all. But if you stop eating food for two months, you'll die, so it is more important to eat properly for your body than to exercise.

Fitness companies have tried to sell their idea of exercise for their own benefit. They are a $2 trillion indus try. So be aware of some of the exercises such as cardio if you are overweight or obese, because they can cause you a heart attack.

So to answer these questions, I will say use common sense

and free style movement. One of my past client's only exercise was dancing, which she enjoyed and helped her to keep her muscles tight. Because when you lose weight your skin has to adjust to your new body sizes, and if you don't incorporate some movement the skin will get slack.

Gardening can give you all the benefits of exercise, and as a side effect can give you fresh food. Another great benefit is that you've improved your environment.

How I can get rid of cravings?

The main reason for cravings is the lack of the important nutrients that are needed in our body, and the poor care of our emotional needs. Sometimes cravings are to fulfill the need for primary food. For example, 80% of the population is unhappy with their own career, and this causes unnecessary stress to the body, and this stress can cause weight gain, unhappiness, and health problems. (It's believed than 95% of all illnesses are either caused by stress or triggered by stress). The primary foods are career, spirituality, relationships, finances, joy, health, creativity & social life.

Let me tell you about one of my clients. She was 295 lbs and in her 30s. I recommended some changes in her diet, a detox, and some movement recommendations, but nothing seemed to work for her. Since I'm a hypnotherapist, I suggested she get hypnotized and she agreed. I always ask my clients to write an essay before the hypnotherapy session, and she did. I did a regression to this life only; I found out that she was the only girl in the family, her mother left with another man, leaving all the kids behind, and that she was the one that had to cook, clean, and also that she was sexually abused by her father and brothers.

When she was in trance, she was screaming, crying and terrified about the incidents. The abuse started at age 10 until she got married. Years later, she was coming out of her house and her younger brother got killed in front of her house.

Before he died, he said I'm sorry.

For her, guilt, shame and anger was a part of her life. For her, gaining weight was a way to keep people from abusing her again. After her first session of hypnotherapy, she changed completely to the point that her husband came to ask me what I did to her. On another occasion her sister came to ask me the same thing. She even told me that she looked like a totally different person. After this, she started losing weight and in two weeks she lost 15 pounds. She move differently, her face lit up, even her cravings went away for good.

So it's time to do some searching if you have cravings. What do you really have cravings for? Be conscious of what you doing, be mindful about your emotional needs and make sure you include all kind of foods into your diet to avoid any cravings.

Why healthy food is so expensive?

Small farmers must spend more money to produce their food. They have to spend more money, more time, and sometimes they lose their entire production of food. The large industries and agriculture companies reduce the costs by putting animals in confined places, and cutting costs on the food given them: lowquality and sometimes waste from other animals' excrement. Their use of pharmaceuticals is greater because their animals get sicker more often. Their plants use tons of pesticides, synthetic fertilizer, and hormones, and sometimes they are genetically modified in order for the large farmers to succeed. Their chickens typically eat excrement of cows; small farmers normally use grains, so it costs more money.

Organic food tends to have more nutrients, due to the rotation of the crops, and animals as well due to the consumption of simple quality grains and grasses. I think our priorities changed over the years, paying millions of dollars to celebrities, sports icons, and so many whose careers are luxurious, that we are forgetting to give credit to the farmers and pay the right amount for food. Good agricultural practice is what we need the most; we have seen around the world the outrageous amount we spend on healthcare.

If you want to get more out of your food, we have to support our farmers that have good practices; we have to pay them a fair price for the food that they produce. So many farmers are walking away for the good practices because they are not cost effective. Some of the farmers even tell their own kids to walk away from the agricultural field because sometimes they can't even cover their own needs and that, my friends, is very sad.

Why healthy food tastes nasty

I know for a fact that good-quality nutritious food tastes great, so many people get confused about what healthy food really means.

Fruits, vegetables, nuts, meat and seeds can make an excellent sources of nutrients. What I have noticed is that a lot of people want to force themselves to eat some foods that are not familiar to their taste buds. We want to incorporate foods from faraway places that our taste buds aren't familiar with. I always recommend eating food that you know, so that you have some sort of relationship with it. Food tastes good to you, so don't follow some food trends. This advice will save you from buying tons of unpleasant-tasting food.

This is one of the main reasons why diets don't work: because they try to incorporate unfamiliar food into the menu.

I don't like all healthy food. Mexicans have a very popular healthy drink made with cactus leaves, pineapple, celery, and water put in a blender. Yes it is very healthy, but it is slimy and I feel like I want to puke. It doesn't mean you are not eating healthy. You can always find another fruit or vegetable that is more desirable to drink. Eat foods you know you like; you can never go wrong with fruits and vegetables in your daily intake of food. Sometimes you can mask the bad flavor with other food that has good flavor. For example, I use blue-green algae in my everyday cooking, such as beans, soups, and many other dishes. I remember once I was talking to another mom from my youngest kid's class, and she was explaining to me that her kids refused to eat anything healthy, so my advice was hide blue-green algae into the foods that they liked the most. Then when I was leaving, my child said I will never eat that nasty thing you say. I just replied don't worry, you will never have to do that (I have given it to my kids all their lives without their knowing).

Here is a good idea. Mix your favorite fruits with foods that you like. For me, I can mix anything with mangoes, berries, apples, pineapple, and grapes, and everything else then tastes so good. This is what always use for my smoothies.

Never again suffer from bad-tasting food. Now you have some ideas for having healthy food without bad taste.

Do carbohydrates make you gain weight?

Not all carbohydrates; fiber can help you to lose weight. But there are carbohydrates such as refined sugar, refined flour, and starches that aren't good for you or your health. These carbohydrates will make you gain weight, mainly fat tissue.

Grains are one of the most common crops that use GMOs; become familiar with the most common applications of genetic modification, the products (and their derivatives) that are most likely to be genetically modified (GMO), mainly used to make the crop resistant to herbicide.

Soybeans —used in variety of foods, fast-food companies use it as filler.
Corn —tortillas, tamales, corn dishes, kernels, and its derivates such as high fructose corn syrup and glucose/

fructose, prevalent in a wide variety of foods in America.
Rapeseed/Canola — cooking oils
Sugar beets
Cotton — the seeds are pressed into cottonseed oil, a common ingredient in vegetable oil and margarine.
Dairy — Cows injected with the hormone rBGH/rBST; possibly fed GM grains and hay.
Papayas, Zucchini

Buy only organic corn, popcorn, and corn chips. Baked goods often have one or more of the common GMO ingredients. Why do we need corn or soy in our bread, snacks, and desserts? It's hard to find mixes to use as well. Some brands avoid GMOs; find those you like and try to stick with them. Again organic is one option; learning how to cook brownies, etc., from scratch with your own organic oils is another.

The U.S. and Canadian governments do not allow manufacturers to label something 100% organic if that food has been genetically modified or been fed genetically modified feed. You may find that organic food is more expensive and different in appearance from conventional products.

Source:http:www.wikihow.com

Grains are to be blame for diseases such as diabetes. One of the main symptoms of diabetes is the enlargement of the abdomen.

We need carbohydrates in order for our body to produce energy. Our body can make energy from proteins. Another smart idea is to use fats as sources of energy, rather than grains. Good fatty foods such as avocados, nuts, seeds, margarine, coconut oil, tallow, fish oil and unrefined extra virgin olive oil can help you to lose weight.

This is one of the most frequent confusions among people.

Grains that are commercially produced have been genetically modified. Also a lot of grains we use are extremely processed. This is why carbohydrates are bad; it's not the grain, it's is all the changes that we make to the grains.

I eat only healthy food, so why am I not losing weight?

First, what do you call healthy? There is so much confusion about the word "healthy". Even professional doctors are confused about nutrition. First we have to make an assessment of nutrition. First we have to make an assessment of what you are eating and your lifestyle, in order for me to determine what is causing you to gain weight.

This is the list of the five causes of gaining weight:

Nutrition

Lack of movement
Chemical toxicity
Stress
Emotional issues

We cannot focus only on nutrition because it's only a portion of the cause of the problem.

What is diabetes type I and diabetes type II?

For us to understand diabetes, we have to know the definition according to the CDC:

What is diabetes?

Diabetes is a disease in which blood glucose levels are above normal. Most of the food we eat is turned into glucose, or sugar, for our bodies to use for energy. The pancreas, an organ that lies near the stomach, makes a hormone called insulin to help glucose get into the cells of our bodies. When you have diabetes, your body either doesn't make enough insulin or can't use its own insulin as well as it should. This causes sugar to build up in your blood.

Diabetes can cause serious health complications including heart disease, blindness, kidney failure, and lower-extremity amputations. Diabetes is the seventh leading cause of death in the United States.

Sources: www.cdc.gov

Symptoms:

Weight loss
Excessive thirst
Frequent urination
Excessive hunger
Dry skin
Feeling tired

Diabetes type I is when your body makes little or no insulin at all.

Most patients are getting insulin shots as a replacement, to restore functioning. Diabetes type I is not always caused by being overweight. There are autoimmune, genetic and environmental factors. Prevention remain elusive.

It usually has more serious side effects if it occurs after having diabetes type II. It doesn't always work like that because some people are born with diabetes type I already, and most of the diabetic kids have type I.

When I was in practice I had a patient who was 19 years old. She was in her first year of college, and as soon as she walked in the office I knew that she had diabetes because her legs were purple black. There were more physicians in the clinic but she was appointed to me. As soon as we started talking, she said I came to this clinic for you to save my legs. For a moment I just looked at her with no answer. The only thing I did was walk out of the room. I went to another empty room, and the first thought in my mind was my daughter. But then my daughter was only 16 and my patient was 19. I asked myself; what would you do if it was your child? I just started crying, having no answers.

Someone asked me what was wrong with me? I told him what the girl just told me, seeing these young people and not being able to help them. Imagine if this was your child.

The reason why the girl was worried about her legs is because so many people with diabetes get amputations, and nowadays younger people have diabetes. In a nutshell, it is when your body stops producing insulin, or if the produced insulin is not enough for your body to function properly.

Diabetes Type II

This is the diabetes that is found mainly in people that are overweight or obese, caused by years of self-abuse, eating junk food, and not exercising. And diabetes type II is fully preventable. I have encountered entire families with diabetes type II, and all of them feel powerless for not preventing this awful disease. But also I noticed that a lot of them never improved their nutrition or their lifestyle.

I had a patient 12 years old, female, 225 pounds. She was only about 5 feet tall and she wanted to lose weight because she wanted to become a model. She was a pretty girl; it was possible. At the time of the intake everything sounded normal, but when I took her blood pressure the reading was 180/110. My first reaction was my blood pressure cuff is not working, so I took another one and that reading was 180/110 again. Then I tried another cuff, and it was the same. So it was not my cuff. This young girl already had high blood pressure. I called her mom and privately told her, and the mother replied, I am not here for you to tell me that my kid is sick. I'm here for you to help my daughter to lose weight because she wants to become a model. I got so mad at her answer that I said to her that if you don't take care of your child now, maybe she's not going to be able to make it, becoming a model.

Here are some of the signs of pre-diabetes: fat around the abdomen, high blood pressure, and being overweight. My 12 year old patient had all the symptoms of a pre-diabetic patient. I have seen so many patients so young with signs of hypoglycemia or prediabetes. Before diabetes was considered an old age diseases, but today so many young adults are being diagnosed.

Get Free Guides:
1.-Are you craving movement
2.- 10 Tips To Lose Weight
3.-Coffee 10 quick Perks

www.healthyhappythinanddietfree.com
Text the word dietfree to 58885

A Doctor that treats illness is a simple doctor, a doctor that prevents illness is a superior doctor.

Georgina Salgado Chavez

CHAPTER 3

When people approach me, their belief is that being overweight or obese is only a cosmetic issue. Some professionals in the field will do anything and everything to make them lose weight, even at the cost of risking the patients' health. I have seen some procedures such as surgeries that have many negative side effects, especially to the digestive system. One treatment that I was amazed that people were even considering is eating the tape worm egg. I have seen patients that have that parasite, and the side effects are horrific, mainly neurological damage. Sometimes desperate people make the wrong choices. I have seen doctors prescribe psychiatric medication for weight loss, with a bunch of negative side effects as well.

What are the side effects of program/procedure?

I always tell my patients it is easy to lose weight, but not all skinny people are healthy. Sometimes I even say something really rude, like if you use drugs such as heroin, cocaine, and even marihuana, it can make you lose weight, but that doesn't mean healthy. Almost everyone agrees with me when I make this comment, so they understand my point of view.

In my 20s I was a loan officer, and a very young couple were my clients. They purchased a house with me. Two years later they came back and wanted to refinance their home. We did the paperwork, and for two weeks the communication was back and forth.

They provided me everything I needed to process the loan; they even paid for the appraisal, and then they disappeared. A month later, the wife told me what happened. The man had neurological problems due to tapeworm eggs. She said that he just forgot everything about himself all of a sudden.

He didn't even recognize her. He had some headaches prior of this incident. He has to be hospitalized because he was really sick. What the doctor told her was that the egg can live there for a very long time before it causes any damage to the brain. Maybe he got parasites from the consumption of pork.

This is one of the main reasons I tell my patients to beware of advice even from doctors; the egg from the tapeworm was prescribed from doctors. If you gain weight over the years, it only makes sense for you to lose weight slowly as well.

What are the side effects of surgery?

Weight loss surgery can be divided into three types:

1. Restrictive procedures to reduce the size of your stomach
2. Mal-absorptive procedures alter the flow from your stomach to your intestine
3. Combination procedures that involve the characteristics of both of the above procedures

We will be focusing on the first option. Gastric bypass surgery is one type of weight loss surgical proceduresthat can be used, and is actually commonly used, to cause significant weight loss for a patient that is exceedingly obese. Gastric bypass surgery is designed to reduce the body's intake of calories. Calorie reduction through this surgery is accomplished in two main ways:

1. After the surgery, the patient's stomach is actually smaller than it was. This means that the patient will feel full faster and it will be easier for the candidate to learn to reduce the amount of food that he/she consumes.

2. Part of the patient's stomach and small intestines are literally bypassed in the food consumption process so that fewer calories are absorbed by the candidate.

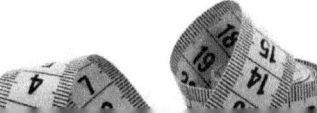

Prior to any successful weight loss operation, the patient's doctor will give the patient a complete medical examination to evaluate the patient's state of overall health. A psychological evaluation will also be undertaken. If at the conclusion of the consultation and evaluation, the doctor does not feel the patient is ready, then the surgery will not be recommended. Should the doctor recommend the procedure, then the patient will receive extensive nutritional counseling before (and after) the surgery.

Gastric bypass surgery is always performed under anesthesia. There are two basic steps to the surgery:

1. The first step in the surgery makes the patient's stomach smaller. The surgeon divides the stomach into a small upper section and a larger bottom section using staples that are like stitches. The top section of the stomach will hold any digested food.

2. After the stomach has been divided, the surgeon connects a section of the small intestine to the pouch. This ensures that the food bypassed the lower portion of the stomach.

Gastric bypass surgery can be performed using a laparoscope. This technique is actually far less invasive than traditional surgery. The incisions are much smaller and therefore are a little less painful and a lot less noticeable, which lowers the risk of large scars and hernias after the procedure. Once the small incisions are made in the abdomen, then the surgeon passes slender surgical instruments through these narrow openings, as well as a camera so that he or she can see the maneuvering of the instruments.

If you have gastric bypass surgery, then you will usually need to stay in the hospital for 4 to 5 days after the doctor performs the surgery on you. Your doctor will approve your discharge to go back home once you are able to do the following:

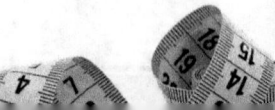

1. Move without too much discomfort
2. Eat liquid and/or pureed food without vomiting it back up
3. No longer require pain medication to be administered by injection

You will remain on liquid or pureed food for several weeks after the surgery. Even after that time, you will feel full very quickly. This is because the new stomach pouch initially only holds a tablespoonful of food. The pouch eventually expands but will generally allow you no more than one cup of food.

According to the Mayo Clinic, here are some side effects. As much as any other major surgery, gastric bypass, bariatric surgery and other weight-loss surgeries pose potential health risks, both in the short term and long term.

Some of the negative side effects of surgical procedures can include:

Excessive bleeding
Infection
Adverse reactions to anesthesia
Blood clots
Lung or breathing problems
Leaks in your gastrointestinal system
Death (rare)

Longer term side effects and complications of weight-loss surgery vary depending on the type of surgery. They can include:

Bowel obstruction
Dumping syndrome, causing diarrhea, nausea or vomiting
Gallstones
Hernias
Low blood sugar (hypoglycemia)

Malnutrition
Stomach perforation

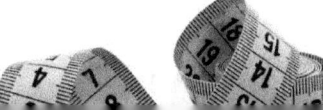

Ulcers
Vomiting
Death (rare)

Source: Mayo Clinic

One of my patients had a part of her stomach removed as a solution for her weight problem. From that point on, she had tons of digestive system issues. She gets frequent nausea, often she has to vomit, pains in the abdomen, and she has trouble eating a variety of foods. She eats very little after the surgery, and she probably is going to live like that the rest of her life. The treatment was recommended and done by a legitimate doctor. He promised she would lose the weight and become healthier, and she accomplished the weight loss without a doubt; but becoming healthier is far from reality.

Get Free Guides:
1.-Are you craving movement
2.- 10 Tips To Lose Weight
3.-Coffee 10 quick Perks

www.healthyhappythinanddietfree.com
Text the word dietfree to 58885

Health is a state of complete physical, mental and social wellbeing, and not merely the absence of disease or infirmity.

~World Health Organization, 1948

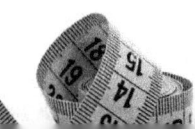

CHAPTER 4

Frequent Myths

Losing weight is very expensive. You have to pay for expensive equipment, expensive food, or it is mandatory to get a membership at the gym.

None of these claims are true. This is what the industry makes you believe. You need to be smart when you are making choices. The industry will look at you as money. Weight management it can be easy, inexpensive and fun, and the price is up to you.

The next time you visit a grocery store, pay attention to the food that it sells that you want to purchase. Read labels, compare the quality of food, such as organic, local, where it comes from, wild, farm-raised, cage-free, etc. Visit places such as farmers' markets to taste the freshness of food compared to the food sold in grocery stores. Buy food from the small farmers. Most of them have good practices similar to the old- fashioned ways.

My father was the principal of a school, but also he was a farmer. Like I said before, my first college field was agriculture. We were very familiar with what's going on and the taste of fresh food.

According to the EPA, here is a list of pesticides that we use in our agriculture fields every day. The worst part of all is that we consume most food with traces of pesticides.

Other examples are available in sources such as Recognition and Management of Pesticide Poisonings.

Organophosphate Pesticides - These pesticides affect the nervous system by disrupting the enzyme that regulates acetylcholine, a neurotransmitter.

Carbamate Pesticides affect the nervous system by disrupting an enzyme that regulates acetylcholine, a neurotransmitter. The enzyme effects are usually reversible. There are several subgroups within the carbamates.

Organochlorine Insecticides were commonly used in the past, but many have been removed from the market due to their health and environmental effects and their persistence (e.g. DDT and chlordane).

Pyrethroid Pesticides were developed as a synthetic version of the naturally occurring pesticide pyrethrin, which is found in chrysanthemums. They have been modified to increase their stability in the environment. Some synthetic pyrethroids are toxic to the nervous system.

Source www.epa.gov

Organic farming, on the other hand, doesn't use pesticides or synthetic fertilizer. It uses mainly waste form another animal such as cows, horses, and goats. Also it is common to use the waste from previous crops. Since the process to produce organically is tedious, a lot of the produce gets loss in the process, and it also takes longer to produce.

Organic food tends to be more nutritious because it is customary to rotate the crops on a yearly basis. This way the soil is rich in nutrients, so you get more for your money at the end of the day.

I tried it all--nothing works, so why bother?

Most people I encounter believe that losing weight is only about calorie intake, exercise, and the amount of food they are consuming. But no one pays attention of the quality of the food that they are putting in their mouth. So many products that are sold in the market as a healthy foods cause weight gain. Here are some examples.

Everyone that I encounter thinks soy is extremely healthy. Here is the truth about soy.

Filled with anti-nutrients, soy contains high levels of phytic acid and phytoestrogens which withdraw nutrients when processed by your body. In the Chinese dynasties the use for soy was for fermented foods, but today soy foods are not fermented to neutralize toxins in soybeans, and are processed in a way that denatures proteins and increases levels of carcinogens. Many of the fast food restaurants use soy as filler for meats due to the cost, because soy is subsidized. Soy has been linked to endocrine disrupters (hormonal imbalances), infertility, breast cancer, hypothyroidism and thyroid cancer. Soy in formula has been linked to autoimmune thyroid disease in infants.

Some of the meat replacements are made mainly with soy, so the next time you use meat replacements, please use whey instead of soy.

Sugar I is added to so many every day products that some of us don't even know the amount of sugar we consume on a daily basis. Unscrupulous companies hide sugar in all kinds of groceries to make it addictive for you to keep buying the products. Most of my clients tell me that they don't consume sugar, but if you dig a little deeper some of them don't even know where sugar is hiding.

Humans love the taste of sweets, but recently sweets come in a more complex form. Today sugar is added to all kinds of groceries, such as tomato paste, baking goods, juices, chips, salad dressing, morning smoothies, barbecue sauce, marinade sauce, cereal, baked beans, yogurt, English muffins, and snack bars, to mention a few. Sugar is addictive and has similar side effects as some illegal drugs. Most of the time addiction starts in childhood, for most of us consume sweets when we show good behavior or during good times such as the celebration of birthday parties, family reunions, Christmas, etc. We relate sweets with something pleasurable, and some people use sweets when they have other emotional needs.

Aspartame is the main ingredient in low calorie, 0 calorie products. It is the technical name for the brand names Nutrasweet, Equal, Spoonful and Equal-measure. Aspartame is highly addictive, so it makes people eat more than usual. The adverse reactions of this product, besides gaining excessive weight, are headaches/ migraine, nausea, numbness, muscle spasms, brain tumors, memory loss, lymphoma, birth defects, diabetes, fibromyalgia, epilepsy, Parkinson's disease, Alzheimer's, mental retardation, fatigue, depression, etc.

Some products in the market that are sold specifically to help you lose weight contain caffeine. They do help you to lose weight, but as we know caffeine can cause endocrine dysfunction (hormonal problems), and also becomes addictive to most consumers.

These are only a few examples of the tricks out there in the market. As you know there are many more out there, so be mindful of what they sell you.

Another common myth is "I can wait until next year to enroll in the program."

I hear this objection so often. Let me ask you something--if your car has a light on, automatically you consider that you have make a trip to the mechanic. Why do you take for granted your own body? The weight is only your body telling you that you need to pay attention to me. I am as important as your car, take care of me.

Your body is not designed to carry that much weight. You get tired easily, develop lower extremity pains, have more difficulty breathing, and impaired to do some activities.

It is important to take care your body even before you become overweight or obese. The most beautiful part of all is that our body is capable of regaining hemostasis, getting back to original form. Don't wait longer if your body becomes sick. It will cost more time and effort on your part.

Do you love anyone? Well, how? First you have to love yourself in order for you to know how love feels. Love means taking care of yourself, then others. Losing weight has so many benefits for you mentally and physically. It is the least that you can do for yourself.

Get Free Guides:
1.-Are you craving movement
2.- 10 Tips To Lose Weight
3.-Coffee 10 quick Perks

www.healthyhappythinanddietfree.com
Text the word dietfree to 58885

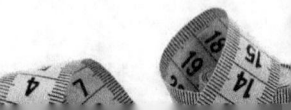

Poor health is not caused by something you don't have;
it's caused by disturbing something that you already have.
Healthy is not something that you need to get, it's
something you have already if you don't disturb it.

~Dean Ornish

CHAPTER 5

If you want to lose weight permanently, you have to know the cause of gaining weight. In this chapter we talk about the causes in detail. Here are the 5 main reasons for gaining weight.

Nutrition

Lack of Movement

Chemical Toxicity

Stress

Emotional issues

Don't worry, you'll get to learn about each cause. I will explain it to make sense out of my claim.

Nutrition

Have you noticed that fad diets rise and fall in popularity like the latest fashions or current pop songs? We've seen (and seen off) the soup diet; the grapefruit diet; the no carbs diet; the only carbs diet, and so on. I remember as a teenager eating only hard boiled eggs for a week! I lost a tons of weight, but I'm never going to do it again! Are you putting your health at risk by following a fad diet?

As a result of experimenting with the latest "food exclusion" diets, many people are actually cutting out entire food groups, leading to nutritional deficiencies, which could be damaging their health! While it may seem that cutting out carbs is great for fast weight loss, there is a very real risk that it will become edgy then start to crave carbs, especially the wrong sort of starchy crabs that are stored as fat. Many people simply give in and become compulsive, but those who hold out can suffer severe side effects. Vitamin B group deficiency is one outcome, leading to fatigue and anxiety.

Did you know the body's main fuel source for energy comes from carbohydrates? Did you know that carbs also are the brain food used to fuel its function? Is it any wonder you carve high-carb, high-sugar snacks when studying hard, problem solving or using a computer? Health professionals advise that eliminating carbs from your diet is counter-productive. A much better strategy is giving your body the right type of carbs it requires.

Others cut out meat when dieting, thinking this is the way to eliminate excess fat from their bodies. By doing so they could be missing out on important vitamins and minerals such as iron, vitamin B12 and zinc. Iron deficiency leads to serious conditions such as anemia.

Protein is an essential building block for the body and is needed for the growth of new cells and tissues. If you don't eat meat it is vital to get adequate protein from other sources such as soy, fish, eggs and chicken.

I have taken so many nutrition classes--holistic nutrition, comparative diets and conventional nutrition. My thinking was that if I learn more I will be able to help my clients/patients more. What I discovered was that everything I've been doing over the years is what we are supposed to be doing, and that was the reason I never gained any weight. Here are my findings:

I will explain what to eat and what not to eat. In a nutshell, more and more people are confused about this topic. Even professionals in the health care system have so many disagreements about what you should and you shouldn't do. I want to ask you a huge favor: read with an open mind. Don't let your perceived understanding get in the way.

Be mindful and listen to the info.

Some examples of the controversies in nutrition are eating meat, raw, vegan, vegetarian, high protein intake (Atkins diet), raw foods, to mention a few. I believe our problem is not the food itself, it is the way that what is being produced is processed that makes it bad or good. For centuries we have been eating meat, fat, vegetables, fruit, nuts, seeds, and roots.

The main problem is the processing of foods, and all the extra things that we are adding to the food to make it last longer and make it look pretty on the shelves.

One of the bigger misconceptions is genetics. So many of my patients/clients tell me it is genetic, I have to be this way because of my genes. Your genome will change due to food or lifestyle (stress).

Only 5% of the health problems we encountr every day are from genetic code. The rest are determined by the food you eat and the lifestyle you choose.

Your gene activity is changed by:

What you eat, drink, breath, and touch

How you feel

What you do

What you think and believe

How you live

What you perceive

Here is an example of magnesium deficiency symptoms.

- ☑ Anxiety and/or Depression ?
- ☑ Poor Digestion ?
- ☑ Headaches / Migraines ?
- ☑ ADD ?
- ☑ Insomnia ?
- ☑ Diabetes / Blood Sugar Imbalances ?
- ☑ Autism ?
- ☑ Heart Palpatations ?
- ☑ Angina ?
- ☑ Constipation ?
- ☑ Anal Spasms ?
- ☑ Fibromyalgia ?
- ☑ CFS; Chronic Fatigue
- ☑ Asthma ?
- ☑ Kidney Stones ?
- ☑ Obesity ?
- ☑ Irritable Bladder ?
- ☑ IBS; Irritable Bowel Syndrome

- ☑ GERD; Acid Reflux ?
- ☑ Sensitivity to Loud Noises ?
- ☑ Irritability or Anxiousness ?
- ☑ Feeling Lethargic or Run Down ?
- ☑ Have Short Term Memory Gaps ?
- ☑ Less Cognitive Function Than Normal ?
- ☑ Occasional Muscular Weakness ?
- ☑ Annoying Muscle Spasms ?
- ☑ Painful Muscle Cramps ?
- ☑ Periodic Muscle Twitching ?
- ☑ Often Tired After A Meal ?
- ☑ Deep Sleep Problems ?
- ☑ Fragile Mental State ?
- ☑ Low Bone Density Issues ?
- ☑ Women; Painful Menstrual Cramps ?
- ☑ Pregnant Woman; Morning Sickness ?
- ☑ Poor Circulation ?
- ☑ Breathing Difficulties ?

Here is a list of what you should be eating:

If you can afford it, organic is better.

Fruits
Vegetables
Nuts
Seeds
Roots
Meats
Poultry
Fish
Dairy

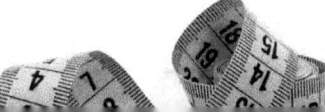

& Fats

Here is what to avoid:

Processed Foods
Refined foods (sugar, salt & flour)
Reduce the intake of grains
Avoid man-made foods at all cost
Avoid foods that say diet, 0 calories, sugar-free

Is this easy? The more you learn about nutrition, the less complicated it is, and you will also understand the claims and controversies. Humans have been eating over 10000 years and it depended on where they lived. They ate what was available.

If you're buying meats, make sure the farmer treats the animal humanely, feeding it grains or grasses, not confining it in small places, and buy free-range and organic if possible.

Fats are needed. Just always keep in mind that our brain is fat, some functions of our body need fat, it is necessary. But go back to what I wrote about fats--unprocessed fats are better than manmade fats, or extremely refined fats. Just stay away from those and you'll be OK.

According to the WHO (World Health Organization), cooking can decrease the amount of people with obesity.

What to cook?

Anything, fresh foods, raw, vegetarian, vegan, canned foods, etc. as long as you begin the process of cooking. This tip alone will make you lose weight.

Avoid fast food restaurants as much as you can. Most of those places tend to use low quality foods, low in nutrients and full of chemicals that your body doesn't need.

Avoid stimulants such as caffeine and pharmaceuticals. Most of the stimulants that have been used for weight loss are highly addictive and have serious side effects to your health. Some patients have the same side effects as a drug addict experiences from illegal drugs. The only difference is that one person went to see a doctor and the other never even got close to a doctor's office.

Go a little farther--eat seasonal, local, fresh and organic for the best outcome, but if you cannot, try at least to cook at home. This can make a huge improvement in your life.

Avoid all kind of man-made foods, processed foods, and food that sits on the shelf for a long period of time. One hint: food spoils very quickly, in a matter of hours. Very few kinds last a couple days, at most.

One great idea for you to lose weight is get into super foods; these foods can provide you with nutrients and fill you up..

You are what you eat; food heals your body, food can change your DNA it is that powerful.

This is mainly Nutrition 101 in a nutshell. You probably you know more than a lot of people who consider themselves experts.

Movement.

We don't really need to exercise, but we need to move and the stretch. You can do simple stuff such as moving around the house, walking around the house, gardening, walking the dogs, going up and down the stairs, dancing, hiking, etc., you get the point. Any movement is better than no movement at all.

Sports medicine recommends 1 ½ hour of intense exercise a week, and 2 ½ hours of mild exercise.

Nothing beats waking up in the morning with the thought of going to the gym to lift weights or jog on the treadmill. After a hard day's work, the gym is one place you don't even want to think about. Sometimes, even the thought of exercising at home with your own equipment can be less than desirable.

Sometimes just trying to get and stay motivated to exercise on a regular basis can be a challenge. No matter how you look at it, exercise can be downright boring and even tedious at times.

So, you may be wondering just how you can get the motivation you need to exercise on a regular basis. If you've been wondering what you can do to make exercise more fun, you'll find some ideas below that just may help to make exercise more fun and a little bit easier.

You can make it fun; get your best friend involved in your daily movement routine.

You can challenge each other, help each other out, keep each other motivated and on track, make each other laugh or just make a game out of your exercise programs.

You can also try something different. If you go to the gym each and every day and use the same piece of equipment or use the same piece of equipment at home, you should try mixing things up. Reverse your routine or just change the order of your exercises.

Go to a city park that has playground equipment and use the slide, climb on the monkey bars, do pull-ups, hang from your knees, just let your imagination guide you. You don't always need to follow a strict routine, just get out there and have fun working your muscles.

An outdoor circuit in the park is also something you can try. There are some parks that have circuit courses set up with a planned course where all you have to do is walk or jog to each station and then follow the instructions. If there isn't a planned course, then you should do a combination of jogging and walking, picking a distance of a couple hundred feet. Jog 100 feet then drop and do a couple of pushups, walk the next 100 feet and then drop to do sit ups.

You can also ride a bike around your neighborhood or hike on a hiking trail. A walk in the park or around your neighborhood is also a great way to get some exercise. Doing yoga in the park or on a beach is also a nice and relaxing way to exercise both your body and your mind.

Playing a competitive sport is also something you can try. A lot of cities have team activities such as softball, volleyball, tennis, soccer, and so on. These types of activities will not only provide you with good exercise but they will also help you to meet new people as well.

When you move, try to picture your muscles getting bigger. Research has shown that if you focus all of your thoughts on the muscles that you are working, they will respond better. Try to watch them work with each repetition as your muscles contract and relax.

As you can tell, there are plenty of ways you can make exercise more fun and interesting. You don't need to follow the same routine day after day, as you can do many other things to get in some exercise.

The important thing is that you should always try to incorporate exercise in any various form into your everyday life and make these habits the kind of habits that will last a lifetime.

Here are the benefits of movement:

Help prevent excess weight

Help maintains weight loss

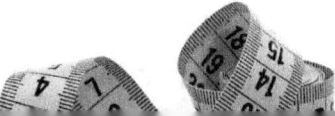

Improve your mood

Improved self esteem

Improved muscle strength

Help you to keep flexible

Help you to keep vitality

Help you to reduce stress

Boost energy

Make you look younger

Help you to sleep better

Combats health conditions and diseases

Puts the spark back into your sex life

Physical activity is a great way to feel better, gain health benefits and have fun. Remember to check with your doctor before starting a new exercise program, especially if you haven't exercised for a long time, have chronic health problems, such as heart disease, diabetes or arthritis, or you have any concerns. Tai Chi, Yoga, Qi Gong, are more than just movement. They also include the breathing portion which can give another round of tons of benefits. Also this type of activity is easy on the joints and helps you with flexibility of the joints and in alleviating pain.

These are some great ideas of what you can do:

A Workout for People Who Don't Want To Work Out

There's good news for people who want to watch their

weight without giving up watching TV. Now there's a new workout for couch potatoes and people who think they're too busy to find time to stay fit.

With time at a premium, many Americans are turning to creative forms of exercise. In a recent survey conducted by Harris Interactive for the North American Spine Society, three out of four people said they used the stairs rather than the elevator at work, 58 percent said they started parking their cars far away in parking lots and almost half reported walking while on the phone.

At the same time, however, 46 percent of people described themselves as couch potatoes--a major contributing factor to being overweight. Many adults say they have procrastinated working out in order to do other activities, such as watching television, sleeping in, doing household chores or working.

Approximately three in four adults say they would exercise more if they could fit it into their daily routines, however, and a majority of adults say they would exercise more often if they could do it at home. Among noncouch potatoes, 80 percent would like to get more exercise, but say they don't have the time.

Meanwhile, more than 4 million Americans suffer disc problems. One out of four Americans over 30 will have recurring back pain, and one in 14 will seek medical care for back or neck pain this year, totaling almost 14 million visits per year. Back pain is the second most common reason that people visit a physician. Back and neck pain result in more lost workdays than any other condition. Due to absenteeism, medical and other related expenses, the cost of back injuries exceeds $80 billion each year in the United States. Exercise is one way to avoid back problems.

That's why it's important to find time to incorporate exercise into your daily routine. In addition to things such as climbing stairs and parking farther away, there are a number of fun ways to make your daily tasks opportunities to exercise:

Feet Alphabet. This exercise can be done anywhere you are sitting, except while driving. It should not be hard to find a place. Simply write the alphabet in the air with each of your feet and ankles. You can do the letters in capitals or small letters and, for that matter, in any language you would like. Doing this two or three times on each ankle will begin to strengthen the ankle and maintain or improve motion.

Doing the Dishes Neck Circles. This exercise is easily done while doing the always fun task of washing the dishes. As you are standing there at the sink, slowly rotate your neck in a clockwise position, trying to extend the tip of your head out as far as possible. After three or four rotations, repeat the exercise in a counter-clockwise position. Remember, these rotations should be done slowly and in a pain-free range of motion. Besides increasing the flexibility of the neck, these exercises can pass the time of doing dishes.

Overhead Laundry Toss. Put the laundry basket directly in front of you and have the washer or dryer directly behind you. Grab a piece or two of dirty clothes, reach over your head slowly and drop the laundry into the washer. Again, start with dry clothes, then progress to wet clothes from the washer into the dryer.

Remote Wrist Lifts. This can be done on any Sunday afternoon watching multiple football games. Simply take the remote control (use the biggest one you have from the pile of remotes) and, while sitting watching your favorite team or movie and with your arm pointing toward the TV, aim the remote at the ceiling, moving your wrist only. Hold it there for 10 seconds, then aim it at the floor, again only moving the wrist. Repeat this three to four times during every commercial. Be careful not to accidentally change the channel when doing this exercise or it may irritate people who are watching TV with you.

These are just some ideas from "The Couch Potato Workout: 101 Exercises You Can Do At Home!" by Joel M. Press, M.D., president of the North American Spine Society and medical director of the Spine and Sports Institute at the Rehabilitation Institute of functional exercises people can do to build strength, balance and flexibility as part of their normal daily routine.

You can still exercise--you just need to sneak in the equivalent in resourceful ways. "The idea is to keep moving," says fitness expert Ann Grandjean, EdD. "Get a cordless phone or put a long cord on your regular phone, and walk when you talk. Find whatever works for you and just move. Park half a mile from the mall and walk. Take the stairs instead of the elevator. Those little, itty-bitty things add up."

Every Stolen Moment Adds Up Lest you think that short bursts of activity have a negligible effect on your fitness program, think again. One study found that women who split their exercise into 10-minute increments were more likely to exercise consistently, and lost more weight after 5 months, than women who exercised for 20 to 40 minutes at a time.

In a landmark study conducted at the University of Virginia, exercise physiologist Glenn Gaesser, PhD, asked men and women to complete 15 10-minute exercise routines a week. After just 21 days, the volunteers' aerobic fitness was equal to that of people 10 to 15 years younger. Their strength, muscular endurance, and flexibility were equal to those of people up to 20 years their junior.

In yet another study, researchers at the Johns Hopkins School of Medicine in Baltimore found that for improving health and fitness in inactive adults, many short bursts of activity are as effective as longer, structured workouts. "It would be useful for people to get out of the all-or-nothing mind-set that unless they exercise for 30 minutes, they're wasting their time," says Gaesser.

Breaking exercise into small chunks on your overscheduled days can also keep your confidence up, says Harold Taylor, time management expert and owner of Harold Taylor Time Consultants in Toronto, who has written extensively on the subject. "Skipping exercise altogether is 'de-motivational'--you feel depressed and guilty," Taylor says. "If you skip it, you tend to figure, 'What's the use? I can't keep up with it anyway.' Yet as long as you make some effort each day, that motivates you onward. Success breeds success."

Keep in mind, though, that short bursts of exercise are meant to supplement, not replace, your regular fitness routine. Here's a roundup of practical ways to work exercise into your day even when you "don't have time to exercise." (You don't have to do them all in 1 day; select what works for you.)

For me, walking the dogs and playing volleyball works fine. You can even make up any freestyle movement that can make you get all the benefits. Last thing: be creative, find something fun and enjoy it.

Chemical Toxicity.

It's believed that chemicals inside your body bind with fat and water, then store in the body. We are bombarded with chemicals in our water, in our food, in our skin care, in our air, in our cleaning supplies, our kitchen, in our soil, everywhere. Living without chemicals is latterly impossible, most of us we have a very amount of chemicals in our body.

The good news is small changes can make a BIG difference!

Here are just some symptoms from toxic foods we eat every day.

Fatigue

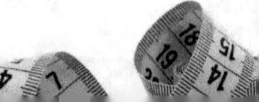

Depression
Excess Weight
Brain Fog
Bloating
Headaches
Joint Pain
Itchy Skin
Sweet Cravings
Sleeplessness
Constipation

People who begin to eliminate toxins from their diet show improved physical, mental and emotional health after the first week!

Where Do Toxins Come From?

Pollution
Metals
Pesticides
Alcohol
Prescription drugs
Food additives
Our normal metabolism
Car exhaust
Intestinal bacteria build-up in our body

Disease thrives in an ACIDIC body. But NOT in an ALKALINE body! You have to have 7.5 pH or better, chemicals tend to turn your body acidic.

Eat alkaline food to:
Rid your body of toxins
Boost your immune function
Prevent parasites, germs and disease
Slow your aging process
Reduce inflammation and body pain
Increase energy and healthy longevity

Alkaline Foods	Acidic Foods
Veggies/leafy greens	Meat/dairy
Whole grains	Refined/Processed
Citrus	Sugar
Fruit	
Water	Drugs/Alcohol
Lemon/ apple cider vinegar	
Green herbal Tea	Soda

Here is a list of some common chemicals used in sprays.

Worst Effects of Air Fresheners.

Methoxychlor: Pesticides that accumulate in fat cells.

Paradichlorobenzene: Causes cancer

Phenol: Flammable, corrosive, and very toxic.

Formaldehyde: Admitted by EPA to be a cause of cancer.

Benzene: Hormone disrupting, can cause birth defects.

1.4 –BCD: Reduces pulmonary function

Naphatalene: Lung irritant; linked to blood, kidney and liver problems.

The color red added to foods has the following side effects: Carcinogenic, increases chance of certain tumors, ADHD in children. The color is found in candy, cereal, desserts, drugs and cosmetics, among other things.

The color yellow is believed to be linked to behavioral problems in children It is found in candy, pharmaceuticals, and cosmetics, among others.

Blue is suspected to cause kidney tumors and is found in

beverages, candy, cereal, gelatin and cosmetics, among others.

Besides what is added to food, there is the packaging plastic used in the food industry. It's believed to be hormone disrupter.

This is only a portion of what chemical toxicity is all about. Before you feed yourself, your family and all your loved ones, please make sure you check. Beware of cosmetics, check your water supplier. Try to avoid as much toxicity as you can.

Stress

According to the medical dictionary, stress is a physical, mental or emotional factor that causes bodily or mental tension. Stresses can be external (from the environment, psychological, or social situations) or internal (illness, or from a medical procedure). Stress can initiate the "fight or flight" response, a complex reaction of neurologic and endocrinologic systems.

Here is another similar definition. Stress is the rate of wear and tear on the body as a result of anxiety, worry, trauma, or exhaustion, from a difficult or challenging situation.

Stress is the body's reaction to primary stimulus: Danger. Danger is perceived by human beings as anything that threatens their mental, emotional, or physical well-being. Under stress, people can experience confusion, loss of control, abnormal behavior, and irrational fear. When the body is threatened with danger, it immediately produces stress hormones.

Stress is a natural part of our body physiology, a mechanism of defense. In medicine it is called the flight or fight response. It prepares us to be ready for an emergency. In school it is explained like this: if you are camping in the middle of the forest and then a bear appears, you going to either fly, meaning run for your life, or fight for your life. At that particular moment your body changes all its physiology, stopping digestion, sending blood to extremities for running or fighting, pupils dilating for you to see better. The heart has to work faster, pumping more blood to areas that need it. This mechanism is OK to have for survival, but it is a problem when we use it continuously. This is when you will have problems with your health.

Drinking or eating stimulants have the same effects. I hear a lot of people mention that if they didn't drink coffee in the morning they couldn't function, because coffee gives them energy. It is not energy, it is your body going into a state of emergency.

What causes stress?

Here is a small list of external and internal factors.

External factors: job, relationships, your home, the physical environment, and all the situations, challenges, difficulties, and expectations you're confronted with on a daily basis.

Internal factors determine your body's ability to respond to, and deal with, the external stress-inducing factors. Internal factors which influence your ability to handle stress include your nutrition, overall health and fitness levels, emotional well-being, and the amount of sleep and rest you get.

Excess stress is a cause of disease and the trigger for almost all illness, and can manifest in physical symptoms or emotional symptoms, and in each individual can be manifested in different ways: anxiety, muscle tension, irritability, headaches, gastrointestinal problems, fatigue, and changed sleeping habits.

The experience of stress is highly individualized. What constitutes overwhelming stress for one person may not be perceived as stress by another. Likewise, the symptoms and signs of poorly managed stress will be different for each person. To avoid stress you would need to avoid life.

Three stages a person goes through in response to situations in life:

Alarm Stage
The body goes into a flight or fight mechanism in response to a situation in life.
For example, a police car puts on its siren behind you.

The Resistance Stage
The body either adapts to the threat or successfully resists it and returns to normal.

The Exhaustion Stage
The body fails to return to normal as in Stage B. This can occur from a prolonged upsetting experience, lowered body resistance, or some form of body malfunction.

In the exhaustion stage, the body overreacts by continuously reacting as if it has to run away or fight. This heightened response causes certain hormones to be released, primarily from the adrenal glands.

The adrenal hormones cause the following changes in the body:

A loss of the ability to digest,
A decrease in circulation to the heart,
A drop in the body's immune defenses by reducing the number of white blood cells,
A drop in oxygen carried to the cells

These reactions over time lead to a host of severe health problems.

Adrenal Stress Hormones:

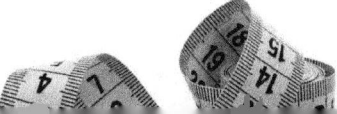

Cortisol: Raises blood sugar and halts the immune response. Adrenaline: Stimulates the heart muscles. Norepinephrine: Constricts the blood vessels, reduces oxygen to cells, inhibits gastrointestinal muscles and increases heart activity.

The adrenal glands can be harmed, not only by stress, but from consuming too much caffeine and sugar.

Vitamin C and certain foods have been found to help repair and maintain the health of the adrenal glands.

The adrenal glands are considered by some authorities to be the "sleep glands", because when these glands are weak, sleep problems often occur.

Some experiments have shown that people with high stress levels tend to develop more colds, and higher incidents of death from heart disease.

The primary symptoms of stress are:

Headaches
Fatigue
Pain and tension in the neck, shoulders or low back
Irritability
Sleep problems
Allergies and sinus problems
Digestive trouble
If you had more than one stress symptom or are having that symptom more than once per month, your body has a stressrelated disorder. Stress affects a person in different areas of their body. If you have a weak neck, stress will affect you in the neck.

If you have a weak stomach, stress can affect you there, causing ulcers, acid reflux, and other digestive troubles. For the body to heal itself and overcome the negative effects of stress, it needs a constant flow of blood and nutrients to all of its tissues and organs.

When there is an interruption to the proper flow of blood and nutrients in the body, you get a weak area. This interruption can be caused by physical trauma from falls or accidents, accumulated tension, chemical stress, anxiety.

How is all this is related to gaining weight? When you release cortisone, your body tends to swell up, so you get puffy, and then your digestive system doesn't work as it should. As I mentioned before, one of the main reasons for weight gain is the inability to excrete the waste. So stress can impair your digestive system function.

What can you do to reduce the harmful effects of stress?

Engage in some form of exercise and relaxation. A recent study followed 40,000 post-menopausal women for 7 years. Those who regularly engaged in moderate activities had a 41% lower death rate than those who did not exercise. California State University found that a 10 minute walk is enough to increase energy, alter mood, and affect a positive outlook for up to 2 hours.

A study done over 7 years by the University of Minnesota involving 12,000 men, found that those who walked or did similar exercise for an average of just 20 minutes a day were 37% less likely to die of coronary disease than those who exercised less than that.

Source: Consumer Reports on Health, April 1998

Laugh. Research conducted at Loma Linda University showed that comedy lowers the body's level of stress, thereby lowering blood pressure and increasing white blood cells and your immunity. Source: Stress: 63 Ways to Relieve Tension and Stay Healthy, Inlander, Charles B., and Moran, C., p.

A study reprinted in the July/August 1995 issue of Men's Health showed toddlers laugh 400 times a day while adults only laugh 15 times.

To reduce the harmful effects of stress, one should eat a healthy diet, exercise regularly, and make sure their body has no interference to the normal flow of blood and energy.

Reduces your intake of sugar Surveys completed by the USDA show that sugar consumption has increased almost annually since 1982. Sources of this sugar commonly include cane and beet sugar – and corn syrup and corn sugar. The cause of this increase is greatly related to added sugars within a wide variety of popular soft drinks and processed junk foods.

Soda consumption has increased dramatically since earlier decades with major soft drink corporations raking in billions of dollars from sales. It's estimated that approximately 33% of added sugar intake is solely from soft drink consumption. Ads for different soda brands are commonly seen in magazines, on billboards, on TV and movies – but what these beverage corporations don't advertise is that sugared soft drinks are the ONLY food that has shown to increase the risk of obesity, which in turn increases the risk for heart disease, stroke, diabetes, cancer, and other diseases. Studies conducted in 2012 concluded that eating too much of sugar may also disrupt one's ability to think clearly due to impaired brain cell signaling.

How much sugar are YOU consuming daily with these common foods?

Here are some negative side effects of sugar:

Sugar can increase your stress levels
Sugar can suppress the immune system.
Sugar interferes with absorption of calcium and magnesium.
Sugar can weaken eyesight.
Sugar can cause hypoglycemia.
Sugar can cause a rapid rise of adrenaline levels in children.

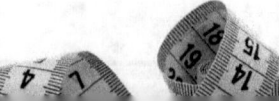

Sugar contributes to obesity.

Sugar can cause arthritis.

Sugar can cause heart disease and emphysema.

Sugar can contribute to osteoporosis.

Sugar can increase cholesterol.

Sugar can lead to both prostate cancer and ovarian cancer.

Sugar can contribute to diabetes.

Sugar can cause cardiovascular disease.

Sugar can make our skin age by changing the structure of collagen.

Sugar can produce a significant rise in triglycerides.

Sugar can increase the body's fluid retention.

Sugar can cause headaches, including migraines.

Sugar can cause depression.

Sugar can contribute to Alzheimer's disease.

In intensive care units, limiting sugar saves lives.

Reduce your stress helps for losing weight, healthy living, and living longer.

Emotional Issues:

You are what you know, not what you don't know.

This means that you act on what you know, regarding your history, how you are thought of by the people that take care of you. Then your mind relates to things in its own way.

Here are some questions that you should ask yourself if you're gaining weight due to emotional issues:

Do you eat when you are anxious?

What do you eat?

What happens when you have cravings?

When do you have the cravings?

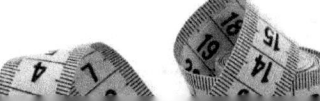

Do you look for food?

Or look for another thing?

When you crave, do you ever check what your soul's needs are?

Are you satisfied with your career?

Are you satisfied with your relationships?

Are you satisfied with your spiritual path?

Do you like creativity?

I had a client who was obese. Everything I tried with him failed. He said something very interesting: the things I like are foods that are wrapped. I asked him which ones? What does that mean? He replied: tacos, burritos, hamburgers, hot dogs, tortas (similar to hamburger), you know. I don't want to eat anything else besides those types of foods, that's the food that I like.

He believed his mom didn't like him; she was always comparing him with her other son, the youngest. He always mentioned that his mom said to him that his brother was a good singer, he was a better student, he was nicer looking, etc. One day I asked him, what are the best memories of your life? He said when I was a kid. Then I asked him what happened then? He replied my mom left me at my grandparents' home; they are the ones that took care of me, raised me, gave a place to live, and fed me. So for me my grandma and grandpa are my parents. Those were the best memories that I had, especially when grandpa just came back from work. He hugged me, then sat on his favorite chair, then he called grandma and said to her, "My old lady, give my son a taco", and my grandma gave me the taco.

You see, for him the relationship with his addiction was something related with his history, which his mind interpreted as something wrapped. He always felt like he was competing his with brother for the love of his mom. He even became a radio celebrity.

Our life story is what most of the time makes the blueprint for our future. Your mind sometimes distorts reality to protect you and to make the best out of it, as a way to keep you safe.

This is one of the main reasons why most of the weight loss programs aren't successful. So few professionals understand human behavior, especially when each of us have our own minds and have a unique road map for ourselves.

I have taken some classes at the Institute for Integrative Nutrition. They teach about primary foods and secondary foods. The primary foods are our necessities of the soul, rather than food for the body. The analogy is basically that we need more than just food; we need food for our soul to fill it out.

The idea here is to have all our necessities in place for our body to gain homeostasis. If we don't have the primary foods and secondary foods in place, our body will be a copy of our instable mind.

This is relevant to the excess weight we get and is one of the main reasons why most of the people don't keep off the weight.

According to Harvard University, happiness can be accomplished by doing certain things on our own. Certain activities can make you produce serotonin and dopamine, chemicals in the brain that make you feel happy. Losing weight also can be accomplished if you do certain activities. Automatically the brain changes the cravings, tending to add more healthy choices automatically.

One thing recommended is to make small changes for the mind to accept as its own; this is why some techniques like EFT, hypnosis, the law of attraction, even praying work very well because they make you tap into areas that are more powerful. I always tell people that all of our power lies in the mind, and that is what makes you or breaks you.

Diets can ruin your relationship with food. This can cause you more weight gain because your brain will play tricks on you over and over. This is one of the main reasons for rebound.

Losing weight can give you tons of benefits as we discussed already. It is for your convenience to lose it the right way, the healthy way. Avoid unscrupulous companies-- the only thing that they in see you is the business aspect.

Conclusion. These are my final recommendations.

Make sure the program that you enroll in is safe.

It should cover all aspects of the problem. It has to include nutrition, something for movement, a detox program should be incorporated (for the removing of chemicals), stress management, and finally a simple way to help the brain to change its bad habits (for emotional issues).

Avoid procedures that can cause you more harm than good in the long run.

Avoid magic pills that can cause negative side-effects or death.

Get into a program as soon as possible; love yourself.

Be patient with the process. It is not how fast you can make it, it is how long you can sustain it.

Love life, enjoy it, and be happy.

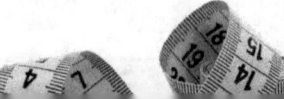

Don't fool yourself about losing weight. If you want to get rid of those extra pounds, jump into a program that is complete, is sustainable, and that you enjoy.

My program that I offer to my clients is simple, easy, affordable and fun. It is something that you can do anywhere you are. No special equipment or special thing is needed to get started.

Get back into activities that you enjoy (like hiking, biking, snorkeling, dancing, etc., you get the point).

Become healthy to enjoy your body, increase your happiness to enjoy your life, and lose weight to have a second chance in life.

Transform your body with ease--start today, don't delay.

Have you been wanting to--

Improve your eating habits?
Understand your body better?
Make your self-care a priority?
Make healthy food choices for you and your loved ones?

Here is a thing to remember: No One Diet Works For Everyone.

I work with my clients to help them create happy, healthy lives in a way that is flexible, fun, and free of denial, and they experience an increase in overall happiness and discipline. Making gradual, lifelong changes enables you to reach your current and future health goals.

Imagine what your life would be like if you had discovered the tools you need for a lifetime of balance. Clear thinking, energy, and excitement every second and accomplishing your goals.

It's rare for someone to get an hour's time to work on improving their health with a trained professional. My programs will provide the tools to personalize your program for a lifetime of health and balance.

It is important that anyone who is losing weight take into consideration the following:

Set and accomplish goals.
Explore new foods.
Understand and reduce cravings.
Increase energy.
Feel better in your body.
Improve personal relationships.

The next time you want enroll in a program, please don't forget to ask questions, and make sure that it is a program that will help you both now and over a long period of time.

Get Free Guides:
1.-Are you craving movement
2.- 10 Tips To Lose Weight
3.-Coffee 10 quick Perks

www.healthyhappythinanddietfree.com
Text the word dietfree to 58885

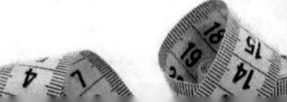

If you have health, you probably will be happy, and if you
have health and happiness, you have all the wealth you
need, even if it is not all you want.

~Elbert Hubbard

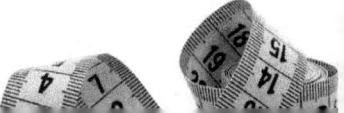